WEIGHT LOSS FOR WOMEN OVER 40

Comprehensive guide to lose weight and look young after 40

Table of Contents

Caution:

It's important to note that individual results may vary and that it's always best to consult a healthcare professional before starting any new diet or exercise program.

Chapter 1:
Understanding the changes in metabolism and hormones during midlife.

Understanding the changes in metabolism and hormones during midlife is an essential step in successful weight loss for women over 40. The human body undergoes significant changes as we age, and these changes can have a significant impact on weight management.

Metabolism refers to the process by which the body converts food into energy. As we age, our metabolism naturally slows down, meaning that we burn fewer calories at rest. This can make it more challenging to maintain a healthy weight, as we may not be able to eat as much as we used to without gaining weight.

Along with a slowing metabolism, women over 40 also experience hormonal changes that can impact weight management. For example, levels of estrogen, the hormone responsible for regulating menstrual cycles and bone health, decrease during menopause. This decrease in estrogen can lead to a reduction in muscle mass and an increase in body fat, making it more challenging to lose weight.

Additionally, changes in the levels of other hormones, such as insulin and cortisol, can also contribute to weight gain during midlife. Insulin is a hormone that regulates blood sugar levels and helps the body store energy as fat. As we age, our bodies may become less sensitive to insulin, leading to elevated levels of insulin in the bloodstream and an increased risk of weight gain. Cortisol, on the other hand, is a hormone produced in response to stress, and elevated cortisol levels can lead to an increase in belly fat and a reduction in muscle mass.

It's important to note that these changes in metabolism and hormones are a natural part of aging and are not always preventable. However, there are steps that women over 40 can take to mitigate their impact on weight management.

For example, regular exercise, especially strength training, can help maintain muscle mass and boost metabolism. A balanced diet that is high in protein and fiber and low in sugar and processed foods can also support weight management. Additionally, stress management techniques, such as meditation and exercise, can help regulate cortisol levels and promote overall health and wellness.

Understanding the changes in metabolism and hormones during midlife is crucial for successful weight loss for women over 40. By taking steps to maintain muscle mass, regulate hormones, and manage stress, women over 40 can increase their chances of achieving and maintaining a healthy weight.

It is also important for women over 40 to seek personalized advice from a healthcare professional, such as a doctor, dietitian, or personal trainer, when it comes to weight loss. They can provide individualized recommendations based on factors such as health history, current health status, and lifestyle. They can also monitor progress and make adjustments to a weight loss plan as needed.

In addition, women over 40 should also be mindful of their nutrient needs, as they may change as they age. For example, the risk of osteoporosis increases after menopause, so it is important to consume enough calcium and vitamin D to support bone health. They may also need to increase their protein intake to support muscle mass and overall health.

It is also important to be mindful of the impact that medications can have on weight management. Many prescription medications, including those for conditions such as high blood pressure and depression, can cause weight gain as a side effect. Women over 40 should discuss their medication regimen with their doctor and consider alternative treatments if necessary.

Finally, it is essential for women over 40 to be patient and consistent with their weight loss efforts. Weight loss at any age takes time and effort, and it is important to not get discouraged by setbacks or slow progress. Instead, it is essential to focus on the long-term goal of maintaining a healthy weight and to celebrate small victories along the way.

Chapter 2:
Importance of a balanced diet with emphasis on nutrient-dense foods.

A balanced diet that is rich in nutrient-dense foods is crucial for weight loss and overall health, particularly for women over 40. As we age, our bodies may require different nutrient needs and may not be able to absorb nutrients as effectively, making it all the more important to focus on a diet that is rich in essential vitamins, minerals, and other nutrients.

Nutrient-dense foods are foods that are high in essential nutrients compared to their calorie content. These foods include fruits, vegetables, lean proteins, whole grains, and healthy fats. They provide the body with the nutrients it needs to function properly, without adding excessive amounts of calories.

Eating a balanced diet that is rich in nutrient-dense foods can also help regulate hormones, support muscle mass, and boost metabolism, all of which are important for weight loss and overall health. For example, protein is essential for building and maintaining muscle mass, which helps boost metabolism and support weight loss. Fiber, found in whole grains and fruits and vegetables, can help regulate hormones and promote feelings of fullness, reducing the risk of overeating.

In addition to consuming nutrient-dense foods, it is also important to limit or avoid foods that are high in added sugars, saturated fats, and sodium. These types of foods are often high in calories and low in essential nutrients, contributing to weight gain and other health problems. For example, high sugar consumption can lead to elevated insulin levels, which can cause weight gain and increase the risk of type 2 diabetes.

It is also important to be mindful of portion sizes when it comes to weight loss. Even healthy foods can contribute to weight gain if consumed in large quantities. A registered dietitian can help provide personalized recommendations for portion sizes based on individual needs and goals.

A balanced diet that is rich in nutrient-dense foods is crucial for weight loss and overall health for women over 40. By focusing on foods that are high in essential nutrients and limiting those that are high in added sugars, saturated fats, and sodium, women over 40 can increase their chances of achieving and maintaining a healthy weight. Consulting a registered dietitian can also be helpful in developing a personalized, nutrient-rich eating plan.

It is also important to note that a balanced diet does not have to be restrictive or boring. There are many delicious and nutritious food options to choose from, and incorporating a variety of nutrient-dense foods into meals and snacks can help ensure that all essential nutrient needs are met.

Incorporating healthy cooking methods, such as baking, grilling, and roasting, can also help keep meals healthy and flavorful. Avoiding processed foods, as well as added sugars and unhealthy fats, is also crucial for promoting a healthy weight and overall health.

Additionally, keeping track of food intake can be helpful in ensuring that a balanced diet is being consumed. This can be done through food journaling, using a food tracking app, or working with a registered dietitian. Keeping track of food intake can also help identify any potential nutrient deficiencies, as well as areas for improvement in the diet.

Incorporating physical activity into a weight loss plan is also essential. Regular exercise can help boost metabolism, support weight loss, and improve overall health. Women over 40 should aim for at least 30 minutes of moderate-intensity physical activity most days of the week. This can include activities such as brisk walking, cycling, swimming, or participating in a fitness class.

A balanced diet that is rich in nutrient-dense foods, combined with regular physical activity and adequate hydration is key for weight loss and overall health for women over 40. By focusing on these important aspects of a healthy lifestyle, women over 40 can increase their chances of achieving and maintaining a healthy weight for years to come.

Chapter 3:
The role of protein in weight loss and maintenance.

Protein is an essential nutrient that plays a crucial role in weight loss and weight maintenance. It is a macronutrient that helps build and repair tissues in the body, and is also involved in various physiological processes such as hormone production, immune function, and the regulation of metabolism.

In terms of weight loss, protein has been shown to be particularly effective in promoting feelings of fullness, reducing overall calorie intake, and supporting weight loss efforts. Studies have shown that increasing protein intake can lead to an automatic reduction in calorie intake, as protein is more satiating than carbohydrates or fat.

Protein also helps to maintain muscle mass during weight loss, which is important for overall health and weight maintenance. As we age, our bodies naturally lose muscle mass, and this can be exacerbated by weight loss if not enough protein is consumed. By consuming adequate protein, women over 40 can help preserve muscle mass and support weight loss efforts.

Incorporating high-protein foods into the diet can also help regulate blood sugar levels and reduce cravings, which is particularly important for women over 40 who may be at increased risk for insulin resistance and other metabolic disorders. High-protein foods include lean meats, poultry, fish, eggs, dairy products, legumes, and nuts and seeds.

It is important to note that protein quality is also an important factor in weight loss and weight maintenance. Consuming high-quality, nutrient-dense protein sources are crucial for overall health and weight loss success. Animal-based protein sources, such as lean meats, poultry, and dairy products, are typically considered to be high-quality protein sources, while plant-based sources of protein, such as legumes, may be lower in certain essential amino acids.

The role of protein in weight loss and weight maintenance is critical. By consuming adequate protein, women over 40 can promote feelings of fullness, reduce overall calorie intake, maintain muscle mass, regulate blood sugar levels, and support weight loss and weight maintenance efforts. Incorporating high-quality, nutrient-dense protein sources into the diet are crucial for overall health and weight loss success.

It is recommended that women over 40 aim for a daily protein intake of at least 1.0-1.5 grams of protein per kilogram of body weight. For example, a woman who weighs 68 kilograms (150 pounds) would need at least 68-102 grams of protein per day. It is important to consult with a healthcare provider or registered dietitian for personalized recommendations based on individual needs and health status.

It is also important to be mindful of portion sizes when incorporating protein into the diet. Consuming large portions of protein-rich foods can still lead to calorie excess and weight gain if not balanced with adequate physical activity and a balanced diet.

Incorporating a variety of high-protein foods into the diet can also help ensure that essential nutrients are consumed. For example, consuming a variety of animal-based protein sources can provide important vitamins and minerals such as iron, calcium, and B vitamins, while incorporating plant-based protein sources can provide additional fiber and phytochemicals that are important for overall health.

In addition to incorporating high-protein foods into the diet, women over 40 may also consider using protein supplements such as whey protein or plant-based protein powders. These supplements can be a convenient way to increase protein intake, but it is important to choose a high-quality product and to not rely solely on protein supplements for meeting protein needs.

The role of protein in weight loss and weight maintenance for women over 40 is critical. By consuming adequate protein, women over 40 can promote feelings of fullness, reduce overall calorie intake, maintain muscle mass, regulate blood sugar levels, and support weight loss and weight maintenance efforts. Incorporating a variety of high-quality, nutrient-dense protein sources into

the diet and being mindful of portion sizes is
crucial for overall health and weight loss success.

Chapter 4:
Importance of hydration and reducing sugar intake.

Hydration and reducing sugar intake are important factors in weight loss and weight maintenance for women over 40. Proper hydration helps regulate metabolism, support energy levels, and promote overall health, while reducing sugar intake can help reduce overall calorie intake and prevent blood sugar spikes.

Hydration is important for maintaining a healthy weight, as dehydration can lead to confusion with hunger and may result in overeating. It is recommended that women over 40 aim to drink at least 8-10 glasses of water per day, and more if they are physically active or in hot climates. It is also important to limit or avoid sugary drinks such as soda, juice, and sports drinks, as these can be high in calories and contribute to weight gain.

In addition to water, herbal teas, coffee, and unsweetened coconut water can also be good sources of hydration. However, it is important to be mindful of added sugar in these beverages, and to choose unsweetened or low-sugar options where possible.

Reducing sugar intake is also an important factor in weight loss and weight maintenance for women over 40. Excess sugar consumption can lead to insulin resistance, weight gain, and an increased risk for chronic diseases such as diabetes and heart disease. To reduce sugar intake, women over 40 can take the following steps:

1. Read nutrition labels: Checking nutrition labels for added sugars can help identify high-sugar foods and drinks that should be limited or avoided.

2. Limit added sugars: Limiting added sugars such as syrups, sweeteners, and table sugar can help reduce overall sugar intake.

3. Choose whole foods: Focusing on eating whole, nutrient-dense foods can help reduce overall sugar intake and support weight loss efforts.

4. Avoid highly processed foods: Processed foods and snacks are often high in added sugars and should be limited or avoided.

5. Reduce sugar cravings: Incorporating protein and healthy fats into the diet can help reduce sugar cravings and prevent overeating.

Hydration and reducing sugar intake are important factors in weight loss and weight maintenance for women over 40. Proper hydration helps regulate metabolism, support energy levels, and promote overall health, while reducing sugar intake can help reduce overall calorie intake, prevent blood sugar spikes, and support weight loss efforts. By incorporating healthy hydration habits and reducing added sugar in the diet, women over 40 can support their weight loss and weight maintenance goals.

It is important to note that reducing sugar intake doesn't mean eliminating all forms of sugar from the diet. Natural sources of sugar such as fruits, vegetables, and dairy products are important sources of nutrients and can be included in a balanced diet. However, it is important to be mindful of portion sizes and to choose low-sugar options where possible.

Incorporating healthy hydration habits and reducing added sugar in the diet can also have other health benefits beyond weight loss. Proper hydration can improve skin health, promote digestion, and support overall health, while reducing added sugar can lower the risk of chronic diseases, improve energy levels, and promote a healthy weight.

Women over 40 may also consider tracking their water and sugar intake to help identify areas for improvement and to monitor progress over time. This can be done through food and water journaling, using a hydration tracking app, or working with a registered dietitian for personalized recommendations.

The importance of hydration and reducing sugar intake in weight loss and weight maintenance for women over 40 cannot be overstated. By incorporating healthy hydration habits and reducing added sugar in the diet, women over 40 can support their weight loss and weight maintenance goals and promote overall health.

Regular monitoring and tracking of water and sugar intake can also help identify areas for improvement and support long-term success.

Chapter 5:
The benefits of strength training for weight loss.

Strength training is an important component of a weight loss program for women over 40. While cardiovascular exercise is essential for burning calories, strength training provides a number of additional benefits that can help support weight loss and promote overall health.

One of the key benefits of strength training is the potential to increase muscle mass. As women age, they naturally lose muscle mass, which can lead to a slower metabolism. Strength training can help slow down or even reverse this process, leading to an increased metabolism and a greater ability to burn calories.

Strength training also has a number of other benefits for weight loss. It can:

1. Improve insulin sensitivity: Strength training has been shown to improve insulin sensitivity, which can help regulate blood sugar levels and support weight loss.

2. Increase bone density: As women age, their
    bones naturally become more fragile and
    prone to injury. Strength training can help
    improve bone density and reduce the risk of
    osteoporosis.

3. Boost confidence and self-esteem: Regular
    strength training can help boost confidence
    and self-esteem, which can have a positive
    impact on overall mental health and well-
    being.

4. Promote overall health: Strength training
    can help improve cardiovascular health,
    reduce the risk of chronic diseases, and
    support overall health and well-being.

It is important to incorporate a variety of strength
training exercises into a weight loss program,
targeting all major muscle groups including the
legs, arms, back, chest, and core. Strength training
exercises can be done using body weight,
resistance bands, weights, or gym equipment, and
can be done at home or in a gym setting.

Women over 40 should start with lighter weights
and gradually increase the weight as they build

strength and improve their form. It is also important to work with a qualified fitness professional or personal trainer to ensure proper form and avoid injury.

It is important for women over 40 to engage in strength training on a regular basis, at least two to three times a week, for maximum benefits. It is also important to incorporate both upper and lower body exercises, as well as exercises that target the core and stabilizing muscles. This helps to create a well-rounded and balanced strength training program.

Additionally, women over 40 can incorporate variety into their strength training routine to prevent boredom and to challenge their muscles in new ways. This can include using different weights, exercises, or equipment, or combining strength training with other forms of exercise such as cardio or yoga.

Along with strength training, it is also important for women over 40 to engage in regular cardiovascular exercise, maintain a balanced diet, and stay hydrated to support their weight loss goals. By taking a comprehensive approach to weight loss, women over 40 can achieve their weight loss goals, improve their overall health, and lead a happier, healthier life.

Strength training plays a critical role in weight loss for women over 40. It can help increase muscle mass, improve insulin sensitivity, boost bone density, and promote overall health and well-being. By incorporating strength training into a comprehensive weight loss program, women over 40 can support their weight loss goals, improve their overall health, and lead a happier, healthier life.

Chapter 6:
The role of sleep in weight management.

Sleep is an essential aspect of weight management and overall health, and women over 40 should prioritize getting enough quality sleep each night. Research has shown that there is a strong connection between sleep and weight, and that insufficient sleep can have a significant impact on weight management.

Lack of sleep can disrupt hormone levels, particularly the hormones leptin and ghrelin. Leptin helps to regulate appetite and energy balance, while ghrelin stimulates appetite. When sleep is disrupted, levels of leptin decrease and levels of ghrelin increase, leading to increased feelings of hunger and decreased feelings of fullness. This can result in overeating and weight gain.

In addition to hormone disruption, lack of sleep can also impact metabolism and energy levels. When we are sleep deprived, our bodies are less efficient at using energy, and our metabolism slows down, making it more difficult to lose weight.

Moreover, sleep deprivation can also impact our ability to make healthy choices and engage in physical activity. When we are tired, we are more likely to make unhealthy food choices, skip physical activity, and engage in sedentary behavior, all of which can contribute to weight gain.

To support weight management, women over 40 should aim to get 7-9 hours of quality sleep each night. This can be achieved by developing healthy sleep habits, such as establishing a regular bedtime routine, reducing screen time before bed, and creating a sleep-conducive environment.

Additionally, it is important to address any sleep disorders, such as sleep apnea, that may be impacting sleep quality. Women over 40 should talk to their healthcare provider if they are having trouble sleeping or if they are feeling excessively tired during the day.

In addition to the above-mentioned effects, sleep can also impact our emotional state and stress levels. When we are sleep deprived, we are more likely to experience feelings of anxiety, irritability, and depression. This can lead to emotional eating, which can contribute to weight gain.

Moreover, chronic stress can increase the release of cortisol, a stress hormone that is associated with weight gain, particularly in the abdominal area. By reducing stress and promoting relaxation through sleep, women over 40 can help regulate cortisol levels and support weight management goals.

In addition to the physical and emotional benefits of sleep, it is also essential for overall health and well-being. Sleep helps to support the immune system, improve memory and cognitive function, and reduce the risk of certain health conditions, such as heart disease, type 2 diabetes, and certain types of cancer.

Chapter 7: Incorporating physical activity into daily routine.

Incorporating physical activity into daily routine is crucial for weight management, especially for women over 40. Physical activity has a number of benefits for weight loss and maintenance, including burning calories, building muscle, and increasing metabolism.

There are many different types of physical activity, including cardiovascular exercise, strength training, and flexibility exercises, each of which provides unique benefits for weight management. Cardiovascular exercise, such as walking, running, or cycling, helps to burn calories and improves cardiovascular health. Strength training, such as lifting weights, can help build muscle and increase metabolism, which can be especially beneficial for women over 40 as they begin to experience age-related muscle loss. Flexibility exercises, such as yoga and Pilates, can help improve posture, reduce stress, and prevent injury.

Incorporating physical activity into daily routine does not have to be time-consuming or involve going to a gym. Simple, low-impact activities, such as walking or doing household chores, can provide significant benefits for weight management. Women over 40 can start by incorporating physical activity into their daily routine for just 10-15 minutes a day, and gradually increasing the duration and intensity as they become more comfortable.

It is important to choose physical activities that are enjoyable and sustainable. Women over 40 may need to make modifications to their physical activity routine as their bodies change, but this does not mean that they need to stop being physically active. There are many low-impact physical activities that are suitable for women over 40, such as water aerobics, tai chi, or gentle yoga.

Incorporating physical activity into daily routine can also provide numerous other health benefits, such as reducing the risk of chronic diseases, improving mood and mental health, and improving bone density.

In addition to its benefits for weight management, physical activity can also help women over 40 maintain independence and mobility as they age. As women enter midlife, they may experience changes in flexibility, balance, and coordination, which can increase the risk of falls and injury. Physical activity can help improve balance, coordination, and flexibility, reducing the risk of falls and injury. It can also help to maintain and build muscle mass, which can be especially important for women over 40 as they begin to experience age-related muscle loss.

Physical activity can also help women over 40 manage stress and improve their mood. Regular physical activity has been shown to reduce symptoms of anxiety and depression, and can help to boost self-esteem and confidence. Additionally, physical activity can help women over 40 maintain their cognitive function and reduce the risk of developing dementia and other age-related cognitive decline.

Incorporating physical activity into daily routine does not have to be expensive or time-consuming. Simple, low-impact activities, such as walking or doing household chores, can provide significant benefits for weight management and overall health. Women over 40 can also consider joining a fitness class, participating in a sport, or simply incorporating physical activity into their daily routine through activities such as gardening, hiking, or cycling.

It is important to consult with a healthcare professional before starting any new physical activity, especially for women over 40 who may have health conditions or other limitations. Women over 40 may also benefit from working with a personal trainer or physical therapist, who can help them create a safe and effective physical activity program that is tailored to their needs and goals.

Chapter 8:
The benefits of a consistent exercise routine.

Consistent exercise is a critical component of weight management and overall health for women over 40. Regular physical activity can help women over 40 lose weight, maintain a healthy weight, and improve overall health and well-being.

One of the main benefits of a consistent exercise routine is that it can help to increase metabolism, which can lead to weight loss and a reduction in body fat. This is because exercise causes the body to burn more calories, both during and after the workout. Regular exercise can also help to increase muscle mass, which can also help to boost metabolism and support weight loss.

In addition to its benefits for weight management, consistent exercise can also help women over 40 maintain and improve their cardiovascular health. Regular physical activity has been shown to reduce the risk of heart disease, stroke, and other cardiovascular conditions, and can help to lower blood pressure, improve cholesterol levels, and support overall cardiovascular health.

Consistent exercise can also help women over 40 to improve their mental health and well-being. Regular physical activity has been shown to reduce symptoms of anxiety and depression, and can help to improve mood, reduce stress, and boost self-esteem and confidence. Additionally, exercise can help women over 40 maintain their cognitive function and reduce the risk of developing dementia and other age-related cognitive decline.

To ensure that exercise is safe and effective, it is important to consult with a healthcare professional before starting a new exercise routine. Women over 40 may also benefit from working with a personal trainer or physical therapist, who can help them create a safe and effective exercise program that is tailored to their needs and goals.

It is important to choose exercises that are enjoyable, sustainable, and safe, and to incorporate a variety of exercises that target different muscle groups and areas of the body. A well-rounded exercise program should include aerobic exercise, such as walking or cycling, as well as strength training, such as weightlifting or bodyweight exercises.

Incorporating mindfulness and stress-management techniques into daily routine.

In addition to exercise and diet, incorporating mindfulness and stress-management techniques into daily routine can be an effective way for women over 40 to support their weight loss goals and improve their overall health and well-being.

Stress can have a negative impact on weight management, as it can lead to overeating and poor food choices, and can also disrupt hormone levels and metabolism. Mindfulness and stress-management techniques can help women over 40 to manage their stress levels and reduce the negative impact of stress on their weight management goals.

There are many different mindfulness and stress-management techniques that women over 40 can incorporate into their daily routine, including meditation, yoga, deep breathing, and journaling. These techniques can help women to reduce stress, improve mood, and increase feelings of calm and relaxation.

Incorporating mindfulness and stress-management techniques into daily routine can also help women over 40 to improve their sleep, as stress and anxiety can interfere with sleep patterns and quality of sleep. By reducing stress and promoting relaxation, mindfulness and stress-management techniques can help women to get the restful sleep they need to support their weight loss goals and overall health and well-being.

Finally, incorporating mindfulness and stress-management techniques into daily routine can help women over 40 to develop a more positive and healthy relationship with food, and can support their efforts to make healthier food choices. By reducing stress and promoting feelings of calm and relaxation, these techniques can help women to make more mindful and intentional food choices, and can support their weight loss goals.

Chapter 9:
Understanding and managing stress to support weight loss.

Stress is a common factor that affects many people in today's fast-paced and demanding world, and it can have a significant impact on weight management, particularly for women over 40. Stress can lead to overeating, poor food choices, and can also disrupt hormone levels and metabolism, making it more difficult to lose weight.

It is important for women over 40 to understand and manage stress to support their weight loss goals. There are several strategies that can help to manage stress and reduce its impact on weight management.

One of the most effective strategies for managing stress is to incorporate mindfulness and stress-management techniques into daily routine. This can include practices such as meditation, yoga, deep breathing, and journaling, which can help to reduce stress, improve mood, and increase feelings of calm and relaxation.

Another strategy for managing stress is to engage in regular physical activity, such as strength training, cardio exercise, and yoga. Exercise can help to reduce stress, improve mood, and increase feelings of well-being, and can also support weight loss by burning calories and boosting metabolism.

It is also important for women over 40 to prioritize self-care, and to make time for activities and hobbies that bring them joy and relaxation. This can include spending time with friends and family, pursuing creative hobbies, or simply taking a relaxing bath or reading a good book.

In addition, it is important for women over 40 to develop healthy sleep habits, as stress and poor sleep can impact weight management and overall health. This can include establishing a consistent bedtime routine, limiting exposure to screens before bedtime, and creating a relaxing sleep environment.

Finally, it is important for women over 40 to seek support from friends, family, and healthcare professionals, as needed. Talking to someone about stress and challenges can help to reduce stress and improve mood, and seeking professional support can help women to develop effective strategies for managing stress and supporting weight loss.

Understanding and managing stress is an important part of supporting weight loss for women over 40. By incorporating mindfulness and stress-management techniques, engaging in physical activity, prioritizing self-care, developing healthy sleep habits, and seeking support as needed, women can effectively manage stress and support their weight loss goals.

Chapter 10:
Importance of tracking progress and adjusting diet and exercise routine accordingly.

Tracking progress is a critical aspect of any weight loss journey, especially for women over 40. Keeping track of progress can help to monitor progress, maintain motivation, and make necessary adjustments to diet and exercise routines.

One of the most effective ways to track progress is to keep a food diary. This can include recording what is eaten, the portion size, and the time of day. Keeping a food diary can help to identify patterns of overeating, unhealthy snacking, and make necessary adjustments to eating habits.

Another important aspect of tracking progress is to regularly measure body weight and body composition. Body weight can be measured using a bathroom scale, while body composition can be measured using tools such as skin fold calipers, bioelectrical impedance, and dual-energy x-ray absorptiometry (DXA). Measuring body weight and composition can help to monitor progress, identify areas where improvements can be made, and make necessary adjustments to diet and exercise routines.

In addition, tracking physical activity and exercise is important in monitoring progress and making necessary adjustments. This can include tracking the type of physical activity, the duration, and the intensity of the exercise. Keeping a record of physical activity can help to identify areas where improvements can be made, and make necessary adjustments to exercise routines.

Tracking progress can also involve monitoring progress in terms of mental and emotional well-being. This can include tracking mood, stress levels, and energy levels. Monitoring progress in terms of mental and emotional well-being can help to identify areas where improvements can be made, and make necessary adjustments to diet, exercise, and self-care routines.

It is also important to set realistic and achievable goals when tracking progress. Women over 40 may not be able to lose weight at the same rate as younger individuals, so setting achievable goals can help to maintain motivation and avoid disappointment. This may involve setting short-term goals, such as losing 1-2 pounds per week, and long-term goals, such as losing a certain amount of weight or reaching a desired body composition.

Another important factor in tracking progress is to seek the support of a healthcare professional. This may include a doctor, dietitian, or personal trainer, who can provide guidance, advice, and support in achieving weight loss goals. They can also help to identify any health conditions that may affect weight loss and provide personalized recommendations to support weight loss and overall health.

It is also important to recognize that weight loss is not a linear process and there may be ups and downs along the way. Plateaus, setbacks, and weight fluctuations are normal and can occur for various reasons, such as stress, hormonal changes, or changes in physical activity levels. It is important to remain patient and persistent, and to make necessary adjustments to diet and exercise routines as needed.

Finally, it is important to celebrate progress and successes along the way. This can include acknowledging small victories, such as reaching a weight loss goal, or trying a new healthy recipe, and recognizing the progress that has been made. Celebrating progress can help to maintain motivation and support successful weight loss.

Chapter 11:
The role of mindfulness and self-care in weight loss.

Mindfulness and self-care are important components in weight loss for women over 40, as they can help to manage stress, improve mood, and foster a positive relationship with food and body image.

Mindfulness is a practice that involves being present in the moment and paying attention to one's thoughts, feelings, and bodily sensations. By practicing mindfulness, individuals can gain a better understanding of their emotional and physical hunger, which can help to reduce overeating and emotional eating. Mindfulness can also help to manage stress, which can have a negative impact on weight loss.

Self-care is another important aspect of weight loss, as it can help to promote overall well-being and support weight loss goals. This can include engaging in activities that promote physical, emotional, and mental health, such as exercise, yoga, meditation, and spending time in nature.

Incorporating self-care practices, such as massage, aromatherapy, and taking time for self-reflection, can also help to manage stress and improve mood. By taking care of one's physical and emotional needs, women can be better equipped to make healthy food choices, stick to a balanced diet, and engage in physical activity.

It is important to recognize that weight loss is not just about losing pounds, but also about improving overall health and well-being. By incorporating mindfulness and self-care practices, women can develop a positive relationship with food and their bodies, which can support weight loss and promote long-term health and wellness.

Additionally, self-care and mindfulness can also help women to maintain their weight loss in the long term. By taking time for self-reflection, women can identify and address any triggers or habits that may be sabotaging their weight loss goals. By engaging in self-care practices, such as yoga and meditation, women can improve their overall mental and emotional well-being, which can help to maintain a healthy weight.

Incorporating self-care and mindfulness into a weight loss plan can also help women to avoid the yo-yo dieting cycle. By developing a positive relationship with food and their bodies, women can make sustainable changes to their diet and exercise routine, which can result in long-term weight loss success.

It is important to remember that weight loss is not a one-size-fits-all process and that incorporating self-care and mindfulness practices may look different for each individual. The key is to find what works best for you and to make it a priority in your weight loss journey.

Incorporating self-care and mindfulness practices into a weight loss plan can help women to overcome obstacles and achieve their goals. By promoting overall well-being and a positive relationship with food and their bodies, women can experience long-term weight loss success and improved health and well-being.

Chapter 12:
Setting realistic and achievable weight loss goals.

Setting realistic and achievable weight loss goals is an important step in the weight loss journey for women over 40. Unrealistic goals can lead to disappointment and frustration, and can cause women to give up on their weight loss journey altogether. On the other hand, setting achievable goals can help to maintain motivation and provide a sense of accomplishment, which can lead to long-term success.

When setting weight loss goals, it is important to consider factors such as age, health status, and activity level. Women over 40 may not be able to lose weight as quickly as they did when they were younger, due to changes in metabolism and hormones. It is recommended that women aim to lose 1 to 2 pounds per week, which is a safe and sustainable rate of weight loss.

It is also important to consider other aspects of health, such as reducing body fat, increasing muscle mass, and improving overall fitness. By focusing on these broader health goals, women can maintain a healthy weight even if they do not reach their desired weight loss goal.

In addition, women should set both short-term and long-term goals. Short-term goals, such as losing 5 pounds in the first month, can help to build momentum and maintain motivation. Long-term goals, such as maintaining a healthy weight for the next 5 years, can provide a larger sense of purpose and help to sustain weight loss over time.

When setting weight loss goals, it is also important to be realistic and flexible. Women may encounter obstacles and challenges along the way, and it is important to be able to adjust their goals as needed. This can include revising a goal weight, changing the rate of weight loss, or incorporating new strategies to help achieve their goals.

It is also important for women to celebrate their successes, no matter how small. This can include acknowledging the small steps they have taken towards their goals, such as increasing physical activity, reducing sugar intake, or making healthier food choices. Recognizing these accomplishments can help to build confidence and maintain motivation, and can serve as a reminder of how far they have come.

Along with setting realistic and achievable goals, it is important for women to have a supportive network of friends, family, or a professional coach. Having a support system can provide encouragement, accountability, and a source of inspiration, which can be particularly helpful during times of challenge or difficulty.

Finally, it is important for women to be patient and persistent in their weight loss journey. Weight loss can be a slow and gradual process, and it is important for women to have a long-term perspective and not be discouraged by setbacks or obstacles. By staying focused on their goals and being consistent in their diet and exercise routine, women can achieve their desired weight loss and maintain a healthy weight in the long term.

In summary, setting realistic and achievable weight loss goals, celebrating successes, having a supportive network, and being patient and persistent are critical components of a successful weight loss journey for women over 40. By focusing on these factors, women can increase their chances of success and maintain a healthy weight in the long term.

Chapter 13:
The benefits of meal prepping and planning.

Meal prepping and planning is a great way for women over 40 to stay on track with their weight loss goals and maintain a healthy lifestyle. By taking the time to plan and prepare meals in advance, women can ensure that they have access to nutritious, calorie-controlled meals whenever they need them.

One of the biggest benefits of meal prepping is convenience. Having meals ready to go in advance makes it much easier to stick to a healthy diet, even on busy days. Women can simply grab a pre-made meal from the fridge, heat it up, and enjoy a nutritious, calorie-controlled meal without having to put in much effort.

Another benefit of meal prepping is the ability to control portion sizes. When women prepare their own meals, they have control over the ingredients and can ensure that they are consuming a balanced and nutritious diet. They can also control portion sizes to help them reach their weight loss goals.

In addition, meal prepping can help women to save time and money. By planning and preparing meals in advance, women can make the most of ingredients they already have on hand, and reduce the need for takeout or fast food. This can not only help to support weight loss, but also save women time and money in the long run.

Meal prepping can help women to develop healthier eating habits. By taking the time to plan and prepare nutritious meals, women can learn to appreciate the taste and benefits of healthy, whole foods. This can help to reduce cravings for unhealthy, processed foods and increase overall health and well-being.

Additionally, meal prepping can also provide a sense of accomplishment and satisfaction. By taking control of their diet and actively working towards their weight loss goals, women can feel proud of their efforts and see tangible progress towards their goals. This can be a powerful motivator to continue making healthy choices in the future.

It's also important to note that meal prepping and planning can be customized to suit each individual's needs and preferences. For example, women can choose to prepare meals for a single day or for an entire week, depending on their schedule and lifestyle. They can also choose to make simple, healthy meals or try out new recipes to keep things interesting.

Chapter 14:
The importance of support and accountability in weight loss.

The support and accountability of others can play a crucial role in weight loss success. This is particularly true for women over 40 who may face unique challenges such as hormonal changes, a slower metabolism, and other health issues that can make weight loss more difficult.

Having a supportive network can provide encouragement, motivation, and a source of inspiration, especially during times of challenge or difficulty. This network can consist of friends, family members, a professional coach, or an online community of individuals who share similar weight loss goals.

One of the benefits of a supportive network is that it can provide accountability. This can help to keep women on track with their diet and exercise routine, even when faced with obstacles or setbacks. Having someone to check in with regularly can also help to keep women motivated, and to remind them of their goals and why they started their weight loss journey in the first place.

In addition to a supportive network, keeping a food and exercise diary can also help to increase accountability and promote weight loss success. This can help women to track their progress, identify areas where they may be struggling, and make necessary adjustments to their diet and exercise routine.

Incorporating healthy habits into daily routine, such as regular physical activity, hydration, and reducing sugar intake, can also provide a sense of accountability and structure, which can support weight loss efforts.

It is important for women to have realistic expectations and to celebrate their successes, no matter how small. This can help to build confidence, maintain motivation, and serve as a reminder of how far they have come.

In summary, support and accountability play a critical role in weight loss success for women over 40. Having a supportive network, tracking progress, and celebrating successes can help to increase accountability and promote weight loss success. By focusing on these factors, women can increase their chances of success and maintain a healthy weight in the long term.

It is also important for women to understand that weight loss is not just about numbers on a scale, but also about overall health and well-being. A supportive network can help women to focus on progress in areas such as increased energy levels, improved sleep, and better overall health, rather than just the number on the scale.

Another benefit of having a supportive network is the exchange of tips and strategies. Women can learn from one another's experiences, and find new and creative ways to overcome challenges and reach their weight loss goals.

Incorporating a variety of activities into a weight loss program, such as strength training, mindfulness, and self-care, can also help to provide a more well-rounded approach to weight loss, and increase the chances of success.

It is important to remember that weight loss is a journey, and not just a destination. A supportive network can provide encouragement and support along the way, and help women to maintain a healthy weight in the long term.

Chapter 15: Understanding and managing emotional eating.

Emotional eating refers to the behavior of eating in response to emotions or feelings, rather than physical hunger. For many women over 40, emotional eating can be a major challenge when trying to lose weight. It is a common and complex issue that can be difficult to overcome without understanding the root cause and developing coping mechanisms.

One of the main causes of emotional eating is stress. Women over 40 may experience a variety of stressors in their lives, such as work, family responsibilities, and health concerns. When stress levels are high, it is common for people to turn to food for comfort. This is because certain foods, such as high-fat and high-sugar foods, can stimulate the release of pleasure-inducing chemicals in the brain, temporarily reducing stress levels.

Another common cause of emotional eating is boredom. Women over 40 may find themselves with more free time as they approach retirement age, and they may not know what to do with it. In this case, they may turn to food as a way to pass the time or distract themselves from feelings of boredom.

To overcome emotional eating, it is important to understand its root causes and develop strategies to manage it. This may involve seeking support from a therapist or counselor, practicing mindfulness and relaxation techniques, finding healthy ways to cope with stress, and developing new hobbies and interests to prevent boredom.

In addition, women over 40 can learn to recognize their triggers and avoid them, or find healthier ways to address them. For example, if a particular food is often associated with emotional eating, women can try to avoid it or choose healthier alternatives when cravings arise. They can also try to eat regularly-scheduled meals and snacks to help regulate their hunger and avoid overeating.

It is also important for women to be kind and gentle with themselves when it comes to emotional eating. This means recognizing that it is a common and normal behavior, and not judging or criticizing themselves for it. Instead, they can focus on making positive changes and learning new strategies for managing stress and emotions.

Emotional eating refers to the tendency to turn to food as a source of comfort, distraction, or stress relief. This type of eating behavior can interfere with weight loss efforts and lead to weight gain over time. It's important to be aware of the triggers that lead to emotional eating, such as boredom, stress, or anxiety, and to find alternative coping mechanisms.

Some strategies that may help manage emotional eating include:

1. Mindfulness: Practicing mindfulness, such as meditation or deep breathing, can help reduce stress and increase awareness of the body's hunger signals.

2. Identifying triggers: Keeping a food journal can help identify patterns in eating behavior

and the triggers that lead to emotional eating.

3. Finding alternatives: Finding alternative activities to cope with emotions, such as taking a walk, reading a book, or practicing yoga, can help reduce the urge to turn to food for comfort.

4. Challenging negative self-talk: Negative self-talk, such as calling oneself "fat" or "stupid," can trigger emotional eating. Challenging these thoughts and replacing them with positive affirmations can help reduce emotional eating.

5. Practicing self-care: Taking time for self-care, such as taking a relaxing bath or getting a massage, can help reduce stress and improve overall well-being, reducing the urge to emotionally eat.

It's important to remember that emotional eating is a common and normal behavior, and that it's possible to overcome it with the right tools and strategies. With patience and persistence, anyone can learn to manage emotional eating and support their weight loss goals.

In conclusion, understanding and managing emotional eating is crucial for women over 40 who want to lose weight and maintain a healthy lifestyle. By identifying the root causes, developing coping mechanisms, and making positive changes, women can overcome this challenge and achieve their weight loss goals.

Chapter 16:
Finding healthy ways to cope with cravings.

Cravings are a normal part of life, but they can be particularly challenging for those trying to lose weight. Understanding cravings and learning to manage them in a healthy way can be a critical component of a successful weight loss journey.

1. Identifying triggers: Understanding what triggers cravings, such as stress, boredom, or specific foods, can help reduce the frequency and intensity of cravings.

2. Eating a balanced diet: Ensuring that your diet is balanced, with an adequate amount of protein, fiber, and healthy fats, can help regulate hunger and reduce cravings.

3. Staying hydrated: Drinking enough water can help reduce hunger and curb cravings.

4. Eating mindfully: Taking the time to savor each bite and tune into hunger and fullness

signals can help reduce overeating and curb cravings.

5. Avoiding deprivation: Depriving yourself of favorite foods can actually increase cravings. Allowing yourself to have a small serving of the food you crave in moderation can help reduce cravings and prevent overeating.

6. Finding alternative sources of satisfaction: Finding alternative sources of satisfaction, such as exercise, hobbies, or social activities, can help reduce the urge to turn to food to meet emotional needs.

7. Mindful snacking: Keeping healthy snacks, such as fruit, nuts, or yogurt, on hand can help reduce the urge to turn to unhealthy junk food when cravings strike.

8. Practicing stress-management techniques: Stress can trigger cravings, especially for sugary and fatty foods. Incorporating stress-management techniques, such as yoga, meditation, or deep breathing, can help reduce stress and curb cravings.

9. Getting enough sleep: Lack of sleep can increase cravings and make it more difficult to resist junk food. Making sure to get enough sleep each night can help regulate hunger hormones and reduce cravings.

10. Moving your body: Regular physical activity can help reduce stress, regulate hormones, and curb cravings.

11. Planning ahead: Having a plan in place for when cravings strike can help reduce the impulse to turn to junk food. Keeping healthy snacks on hand or having a backup plan for a healthy alternative can help overcome cravings.

12. Seeking support: Surrounding yourself with supportive friends and family can provide the encouragement and accountability needed to resist cravings and achieve weight loss goals.

13. Seeking professional help: For some people, cravings can be a sign of an underlying issue, such as an eating disorder or food addiction. Seeking professional help from a

therapist or nutritionist can help address these deeper issues and provide a personalized approach to managing cravings.

Remember, it's okay to have cravings, and it's important to find healthy ways to cope with them. With practice and patience, anyone can learn to manage cravings and achieve their weight loss goals.

Chapter 17:
The benefits of resistance training for weight loss.

Resistance training, also known as strength training, is a type of exercise that involves using weights or resistance to strengthen and build muscle. Resistance training can play a key role in weight loss for women over 40, as it provides numerous health benefits beyond just burning calories during a workout.

1. Increases metabolism: Resistance training can increase muscle mass, which in turn can boost metabolism. The more muscle mass you have, the more calories you'll burn at rest. This means you'll continue to burn calories even after your workout is over.

2. Builds muscle: As women age, they tend to lose muscle mass. Resistance training helps to build and maintain muscle mass, which can help prevent age-related muscle loss and maintain a healthy weight.

3. Burns fat: Resistance training can help burn fat by building muscle and increasing metabolism. This can lead to a reduction in overall body fat, particularly in stubborn areas such as the stomach, hips, and thighs.

4. Improves bone density: Resistance training can help improve bone density, which is important for women over 40 who are at an increased risk of osteoporosis.

5. Enhances functional fitness: Resistance training can help improve balance, stability, and coordination, which can be especially important for women over 40 as they age.

6. Boosts confidence: Resistance training can help improve body image and self-confidence, which can be especially important for women over 40 who may be experiencing changes in their body due to aging or menopause.

7. Increases endurance: Resistance training can help increase endurance, which can help improve overall physical fitness and make it easier to participate in physical

activities such as hiking, cycling, or playing with children or grandchildren.

8. Reduces risk of chronic disease: Resistance training can help reduce the risk of chronic diseases such as heart disease, type 2 diabetes, and certain types of cancer.

It's important to consult with a doctor or personal trainer before starting a resistance training program, especially if you have any medical conditions or are new to exercise. Resistance training should be done in conjunction with a balanced diet and regular physical activity for best results.

Resistance training is an effective way for women over 40 to lose weight and maintain weight loss. This type of exercise involves using weights or resistance bands to build muscle, which in turn increases the body's metabolism. Building muscle mass through resistance training can also improve bone density and reduce the risk of osteoporosis, a common concern for women as they age.

Incorporating resistance training into a weight loss routine can also help to shape and tone the body, resulting in a more defined and toned appearance. Resistance training is particularly effective in targeting specific areas of the body, such as the arms, legs, and abdominal muscles, allowing women to target specific areas they may want to improve.

Resistance training can also be done in a variety of ways, such as through weightlifting, bodyweight exercises, and the use of resistance bands. This allows women to find a type of resistance training that suits their individual preferences and needs. Additionally, resistance training can be done at home, in a gym, or even while traveling, making it an accessible form of exercise for women of all lifestyles.

It is important to start with a gradual progression in weight and intensity when incorporating resistance training into a weight loss routine. Women over 40 should also seek guidance from a qualified personal trainer or physical therapist to ensure proper form and technique, and to avoid injury.

Chapter 18:
The importance of stretching and recovery after exercise.

Stretching and recovery after exercise are important components of any fitness routine, and they play a crucial role in weight loss for women over 40. When the body is subjected to intense physical activity, it is common for the muscles to become tight and stiff, which can lead to pain, discomfort, and injury. Regular stretching helps to prevent these issues by increasing flexibility and improving range of motion.

There are many different types of stretching, including dynamic stretching, which involves moving the body through a range of motion, and static stretching, which involves holding a stretch for a period of time. Women over 40 are advised to engage in a variety of stretching activities to ensure that all muscle groups are targeted, including stretching for the legs, hips, back, arms, and neck.

In addition to stretching, recovery is also important after exercise. This involves engaging in activities that help the body to repair and regenerate, such as rest, hydration, and good nutrition. Women over 40 should aim to get adequate sleep and eat a balanced diet that provides the necessary nutrients to support recovery and promote overall health.

Incorporating stretching and recovery into a fitness routine can also have mental health benefits, as it can help to reduce stress and improve feelings of well-being. This is especially important for women over 40, who may experience hormonal changes and other challenges during this time.

Overall, incorporating stretching and recovery into a weight loss routine is an important step in promoting healthy and sustainable weight loss for women over 40. By prioritizing these activities, women can support their overall health and well-being, and achieve their weight loss goals in a safe and effective manner.

Stretching and recovery after exercise are critical components of a well-rounded fitness routine, especially for women over 40. Stretching helps improve flexibility and reduces the risk of injury during physical activity. It also promotes better posture, helps relieve muscle tension, and increases blood flow to the muscles, which can enhance recovery after a workout.

Recovery is an essential part of the weight loss process, as it helps repair and rebuild muscle tissue damaged during exercise. This can lead to improved muscle strength and tone, which in turn can increase metabolism, helping to support weight loss.

There are several ways to incorporate stretching and recovery into your routine, including yoga, foam rolling, and stretching after a workout. Yoga can be especially beneficial for women over 40, as it helps improve flexibility, balance, and stability, while also reducing stress and promoting relaxation.

Foam rolling is another excellent way to promote recovery and reduce muscle soreness. This form of self-massage can help improve circulation, reduce muscle tension, and release tightness in the fascia, which can lead to improved flexibility and range of motion.

Stretching after a workout is also important, as it can help reduce muscle soreness and promote recovery. Simple stretches, such as calf raises, quad stretches, and hamstring stretches, can help improve flexibility and reduce muscle tension.

Incorporating stretching and recovery into your routine can help ensure that you're able to maintain your fitness goals, avoid injury, and support weight loss in a sustainable way.

Chapter 19:
The benefits of a fiber-rich diet for weight loss.

The human body requires a variety of nutrients to function properly, and fiber is one of the most important of these. Fiber is a type of carbohydrate that cannot be digested by the human body, and as a result, it travels through the digestive system largely intact. This makes fiber an important part of a weight loss diet because it helps regulate the digestive system and promotes feelings of fullness and satisfaction after eating.

For women over 40, incorporating fiber into their diet can be especially important as they face changes in metabolism and hormonal balance. A diet high in fiber can help regulate blood sugar levels, which can help control cravings and hunger. It can also help support digestive health, which can be particularly important as women experience changes in their hormones during this stage of life.

Fiber-rich foods include whole grains, fruits, vegetables, nuts, and legumes. These foods are also nutrient-dense, which means they are high in essential vitamins, minerals, and antioxidants that the body needs to function at its best.

Incorporating fiber into the diet can be as simple as making small, gradual changes, such as choosing whole grain bread instead of white bread, snacking on raw fruits and vegetables instead of processed snacks, and adding beans to salads and soups.

In addition to supporting weight loss, a fiber-rich diet can also help reduce the risk of various health conditions, such as heart disease, stroke, and certain types of cancer. It can also help regulate bowel movements, reduce inflammation, and support overall health and wellness.

For women over 40 who are looking to lose weight, incorporating fiber into their diet is an important step towards achieving their goals. By focusing on nutrient-dense, fiber-rich foods, they can support their health, regulate their digestive system, and achieve their desired weight loss outcomes in a healthy and sustainable way.

Fiber is an important nutrient that plays a significant role in weight management. A fiber-rich diet is beneficial for weight loss for several reasons. Firstly, fiber helps to promote feelings of fullness, reducing the overall caloric intake. This is because fiber takes longer to digest, which means that it remains in the digestive system for longer, providing a sense of satiety and reducing the urge to snack between meals.

In addition to promoting feelings of fullness, fiber also slows down the absorption of sugar and other nutrients, preventing spikes in blood sugar levels and reducing the risk of type 2 diabetes. This is particularly important for women over 40, who are more likely to be at risk of developing diabetes due to hormonal changes and a slower metabolism.

Furthermore, fiber helps to regulate bowel movements and prevent constipation, which can lead to bloating and a feeling of sluggishness. This is particularly important for weight loss, as bloating can make it difficult to accurately assess progress and it can be discouraging when the scale does not move as expected.

Finally, fiber helps to feed the beneficial gut bacteria, promoting a healthy gut microbiome. A healthy gut microbiome is important for weight loss, as it can influence hormones and metabolism, as well as reducing inflammation and improving gut health.

To incorporate more fiber into the diet, women over 40 can focus on eating a variety of high-fiber foods, such as whole grains, fruits, vegetables, legumes, and nuts and seeds. It is important to gradually increase fiber intake, as too much too quickly can lead to digestive discomfort. In addition, it is important to drink plenty of water when consuming fiber, as this will help to prevent constipation and promote regular bowel movements.

Chapter 20:
Incorporating healthy habits into daily routine for long-term success.

Incorporating healthy habits into daily routine for long-term success is a key aspect of sustainable weight loss. This chapter will discuss the importance of developing and maintaining healthy habits that support weight loss and overall well-being.

Studies have shown that forming habits can take anywhere from 18 to 254 days, but once they are established, they become automatic and require minimal effort to maintain. This makes them an ideal tool for maintaining weight loss over the long term.

Here are some healthy habits that can be incorporated into daily routine to support weight loss:

1. Eating regularly: Eating regular, balanced meals and snacks can help regulate metabolism, control hunger and prevent overeating.

2. Drinking plenty of water: Staying hydrated is crucial for weight loss, as it helps to flush out toxins and maintain a healthy metabolism. Aim to drink at least 8 glasses of water per day.

3. Getting enough sleep: Sleep is crucial for weight loss, as it helps to regulate hormones that control hunger and metabolism. Aim for 7-9 hours of quality sleep each night.

4. Incorporating physical activity: Regular exercise is essential for weight loss and overall health. Aim to incorporate 30 minutes of moderate physical activity into your daily routine.

5. Practicing stress management: Chronic stress can increase cortisol levels and lead to weight gain. Incorporating stress-management techniques, such as mindfulness, meditation, and yoga, can help to reduce stress and support weight loss.

6. Keeping track of progress: Keeping track of progress through journaling, tracking food

and exercise, or using a Smartphone app can help to keep you motivated and on track with your weight loss goals.

7. Surrounding yourself with supportive people: Surrounding yourself with friends and family who support your weight loss goals can provide the encouragement and accountability needed to achieve long-term success.

Maintaining a healthy lifestyle is not just about losing weight, but it's about creating a sustainable routine that will improve your overall health and well-being. Incorporating healthy habits into your daily routine can be challenging, especially if you're starting from scratch. However, the benefits of a healthy lifestyle are numerous, and by making gradual changes, you can achieve long-term success.

One healthy habit you can incorporate into your daily routine is to eat more fiber-rich foods. Fiber is an essential nutrient that helps you feel full, regulates digestion, and reduces the risk of various health issues, such as heart disease and diabetes. A fiber-rich diet can also help you lose weight, as fiber-rich foods take longer to digest, keeping you feeling full for longer periods of time.

Staying hydrated is also important for weight loss and overall health. Water helps regulate body temperature, transport nutrients, and remove waste. It's also essential for digestion and metabolism. By drinking plenty of water, you can help your body function at its best and reduce the risk of dehydration, which can lead to fatigue, headaches, and other health issues.

Finally, it's important to take care of your body after exercise, whether that's through stretching, recovery exercises, or rest. Stretching is a great way to improve flexibility, reduce the risk of injury, and increase blood flow to your muscles. Additionally, recovery exercises can help your body repair itself after intense exercise, reducing the risk of injury and soreness. By taking care of your body after exercise, you can ensure you're ready to tackle your next workout.

In conclusion, incorporating healthy habits into your daily routine can be challenging, but the benefits are numerous. Whether it's eating a fiber-rich diet, staying hydrated, or taking care of your body after exercise, these habits can help you achieve long-term success in your weight loss journey. By taking small steps and making gradual changes, you can create a healthy and sustainable lifestyle that will improve your overall health and well-being.

Chapter 21:
The role of protein in maintaining muscle mass during weight loss.

Protein is a vital nutrient that plays a critical role in maintaining muscle mass during weight loss. As women over 40 lose weight, it is essential to ensure that they are not losing muscle mass along with fat. Losing muscle mass can slow down the metabolism, making it harder to maintain weight loss in the long run. This is why incorporating protein into the diet is crucial for successful weight loss.

Protein is essential for building and repairing muscle tissue, and it also helps to keep the metabolism running efficiently. It takes more energy to digest protein than it does to digest carbohydrates or fats, so eating protein-rich foods can help increase the metabolism and burn more calories.

Research has shown that consuming adequate amounts of protein can help to preserve muscle mass during weight loss. This is especially important for women over 40, who may be more susceptible to muscle loss due to hormonal changes and the natural aging process.

Incorporating protein-rich foods into each meal and snack can help women over 40 maintain muscle mass while losing weight. Good sources of protein include lean meats, poultry, fish, eggs, dairy products, and plant-based protein sources such as beans, lentils, and tofu.

It is also important to note that protein should be consumed in moderation as part of a balanced diet. Consuming too much protein can lead to health issues, such as kidney damage and elevated levels of cholesterol.

It is recommended that women over 40 consume 1.0-1.5 grams of protein per kilogram of body weight per day to maintain muscle mass during weight loss. This can be achieved by incorporating protein-rich foods into their diet such as lean meats, poultry, fish, dairy products, eggs, and legumes. It is also important to vary their protein sources to ensure they are getting all of the essential amino acids needed for optimal muscle health.

Incorporating protein into each meal and snack can also help keep them feeling full and satisfied, reducing the risk of overeating and promoting weight loss. Additionally, consuming protein after exercise can help repair and rebuild muscle tissue, allowing women over 40 to maximize the benefits of their workouts.

Chapter 22:
Understanding and avoiding common weight loss pitfalls.

Weight loss can be a challenging journey, and it's important to understand common pitfalls to avoid them. Some common pitfalls include:

1. Yo-yo dieting: Rapid weight loss followed by weight gain can lead to a cycle of yo-yo dieting, which can be harmful to both physical and mental health.

2. Fad diets: Diets that promise quick and easy weight loss are often not sustainable and can lead to the yo-yo dieting cycle.

3. Restrictive diets: Restrictive diets can lead to feelings of deprivation, which can cause individuals to fall off the wagon and give into cravings.

4. Lack of progress: It can be disheartening to not see progress despite following a diet and exercise routine, which can lead to feelings of frustration and discouragement.

5. Lack of support: Without proper support and accountability, it can be challenging to stay on track with a weight loss journey.

6. Underestimating calorie intake: Many individuals underestimate the number of calories they consume, which can make it difficult to lose weight.

7. Skipping meals: Skipping meals can lead to feelings of hunger and decreased energy levels, which can cause individuals to give into cravings.

8. Focusing on scale weight: The number on the scale can be deceiving and doesn't take into account changes in muscle mass, water weight, and body composition.

9. Not adjusting diet and exercise routine: Without adjusting diet and exercise routine based on progress and goals, weight loss progress can plateau or slow down.

By being aware of these common pitfalls, individuals can work to avoid them and set themselves up for success in their weight loss journey. Additionally, it's important to remember that weight loss is a journey and progress may not happen overnight. It's important to be patient and persistent, and to celebrate small victories along the way.

Weight loss can be a challenging journey, especially for women over 40 who may be facing changes in metabolism and hormones. However, it is possible to lose weight and keep it off by making lifestyle changes and incorporating healthy habits into daily routines. One of the common pitfalls that people often fall into is the all-or-nothing mindset. This can be tempting, especially in the beginning stages of weight loss when there is a lot of enthusiasm. People may go from eating poorly to eating only healthy foods, and from being sedentary to working out intensely every day. But this approach is unsustainable, and it can often lead to burnout and giving up on weight loss altogether. A better approach is to start small and make gradual changes, such as drinking more water, reducing sugar intake, and incorporating physical activity into daily routines. This way, weight loss becomes a sustainable and achievable goal.

Chapter 23:
The importance of a well-rounded fitness routine for weight loss.

Weight loss is a complex process that involves multiple factors, including diet, exercise, sleep, and stress management. While diet and exercise are the most critical components of a weight loss plan, a well-rounded fitness routine can greatly improve weight loss outcomes.

A well-rounded fitness routine should include a mix of cardio and strength training exercises, as well as flexibility and recovery activities. Cardio exercises such as running, cycling, or swimming can help burn calories, increase heart rate, and improve cardiovascular health. Strength training exercises, on the other hand, can help build muscle, increase metabolism, and maintain muscle mass during weight loss.

Incorporating flexibility exercises such as stretching or yoga can help improve posture, reduce stress, and prevent injury. Additionally, recovery activities such as foam rolling or massage can help reduce muscle soreness, improve flexibility, and promote healing after exercise.

It's also important to vary your fitness routine to prevent boredom and promote progress. For example, you can switch between different types of cardio exercises or try new strength training exercises to target different muscle groups.

Having a well-rounded fitness routine can also provide numerous physical and mental health benefits beyond weight loss. Regular exercise can help reduce the risk of chronic diseases such as heart disease, diabetes, and certain types of cancer. Exercise can also improve mood, reduce stress, and increase energy levels.

A well-rounded fitness routine is important for weight loss because it helps to target different areas of the body, improve overall fitness, and prevent boredom. By incorporating a variety of exercises, such as cardio, strength training, and flexibility exercises, individuals can maximize the benefits of their workout routine.

Cardio exercises, such as running, cycling, or swimming, are great for improving cardiovascular health and burning calories. They also increase heart rate, which can help boost metabolism. Strength training, on the other hand, is important for building and maintaining muscle mass, which is important for weight loss because muscle tissue burns more calories than fat tissue. Resistance exercises, such as weight lifting or bodyweight exercises, can help increase muscle mass and promote weight loss.

In addition to cardio and strength training, it is important to include stretching and flexibility exercises in a well-rounded fitness routine. These types of exercises help to improve range of motion, reduce muscle tightness, and prevent injury. Stretching also promotes relaxation and stress relief, which can be beneficial for individuals who are trying to manage their weight.

Finally, incorporating a variety of exercises into a fitness routine can help prevent boredom, which is a common reason why people stop working out. By mixing things up and trying new activities, individuals can keep their fitness routine exciting and motivating.

Chapter 24:
The role of community and support in weight loss.

The role of community and support in weight loss is a crucial aspect of weight management and can greatly impact one's success. When people are trying to lose weight, it can be a challenging and overwhelming process, and having a supportive community can make a significant difference. Support from friends, family, and like-minded individuals can provide encouragement, motivation, and accountability. Additionally, being part of a community can help people feel less isolated and more connected, which can be especially beneficial for those who are struggling with emotional eating or other weight-related issues.

Research has shown that people who have social support are more likely to stick to their weight loss goals and maintain their weight loss over time. This support can come in many forms, such as participating in a weight loss group, joining a fitness class, or having a workout buddy. Having someone to share experiences, successes, and setbacks with can provide a sense of comfort and validation, and can also lead to new relationships and a stronger sense of community.

In addition to social support, having a sense of accountability can also be beneficial. When people have someone who is counting on them to show up for a workout or make healthier choices, they are more likely to follow through with their weight loss goals. This can come in the form of a workout partner, a coach, or even a social media group where people can share their progress and get feedback and encouragement from others.

Community and support also play a role in reducing stress, which can be a major factor in weight gain and weight loss resistance. When people are under stress, they are more likely to engage in emotional eating and make unhealthy food choices. Having a supportive community can help individuals manage stress in healthy ways and provide a sense of comfort and security.

Community and support play a significant role in weight loss and can make the journey much easier and more manageable. When individuals embark on a weight loss journey, it can be difficult to maintain their motivation and commitment without the help of others. This is why having a supportive community can be extremely beneficial.

One of the main benefits of having a supportive community is the accountability it provides. When individuals have a support system, they are more likely to stick to their diet and exercise routine because they feel accountable to their friends and family. Furthermore, having a community can also provide a source of encouragement and motivation, which can help individuals stay on track even when they encounter setbacks or obstacles.

Having a community can also help individuals manage their emotions and reduce stress levels, which is critical in weight loss. When people are undergoing weight loss, they may experience feelings of stress, anxiety, and frustration, which can trigger emotional eating and sabotage their efforts. A supportive community can provide a safe and supportive environment in which individuals can express their feelings and receive the support they need.

Additionally, a supportive community can also provide individuals with valuable information, resources, and advice on weight loss and healthy living. For example, community members can share their experiences, tips, and advice on diet and exercise, which can help individuals make better choices and achieve their goals more efficiently.

Moreover, participating in community events, such as fitness classes, weight loss challenges, or outdoor activities, can provide individuals with a fun and enjoyable way to stay active and motivated. These activities can also provide individuals with an opportunity to make new friends, who may become a part of their support system.

Chapter 25:
Celebrating progress and learning from setbacks to maintain a healthy weight long-term.

The process of losing weight and maintaining a healthy weight is often a long-term journey that requires persistence, dedication, and the development of healthy habits. Achieving a healthy weight is not only about making changes to diet and exercise, but also about creating a supportive environment, managing stress, and maintaining a positive outlook. In this chapter, we will explore the importance of celebrating progress and learning from setbacks as part of a long-term weight loss journey.

One of the key aspects of weight loss is tracking progress and celebrating the small victories along the way. Whether it's losing a few pounds, fitting into a smaller size, or simply feeling better, acknowledging these accomplishments can provide motivation to continue making healthy choices. This sense of accomplishment can also help maintain a positive outlook and keep the focus on the long-term goal.

However, setbacks are an inevitable part of the weight loss journey, and it's important to be prepared for them. Rather than becoming discouraged by setbacks, it's important to view them as opportunities for growth and learning. By understanding the reasons for setbacks, such as a lapse in healthy habits or a period of stress, individuals can make adjustments and refocus their efforts.

Incorporating self-care and mindfulness can also help maintain a positive outlook and resilience during setbacks. This can include practices such as yoga, meditation, or taking time for hobbies and activities that bring joy.

The role of community and support cannot be overstated in the weight loss journey. Having friends, family, or a support group can provide encouragement and accountability, and can help individuals stay motivated and on track. Celebrating progress and learning from setbacks as part of a supportive community can make the weight loss journey a more enjoyable and rewarding experience.

Celebrating progress and learning from setbacks is an important part of the weight loss journey. This chapter focuses on the importance of recognizing and appreciating small wins and using them to motivate you towards your long-term goal. It also emphasizes the importance of not letting setbacks discourage you, but rather using them as learning opportunities to improve your journey.

Incorporating regular self-reflection and self-awareness can help you understand why you may have experienced a setback, and what you can do to prevent similar situations in the future. This can help you stay on track and maintain your weight loss progress.

It's also important to understand that weight loss is not always a linear process and that it's normal to experience ups and downs along the way. By celebrating progress, learning from setbacks and focusing on the bigger picture, you can stay motivated and continue making progress towards your goals.

In addition, having a supportive community and forming healthy relationships with those around you can help you stay accountable and on track with your weight loss journey. Whether it's a group of friends, a gym buddy or a support group, having people to turn to who understand and support your journey can be incredibly beneficial.

Finally, it's important to recognize and celebrate your achievements, both big and small. This can help you stay motivated and stay committed to your weight loss journey, even during difficult times.

Overall, the chapter highlights the importance of having a positive outlook, being self-aware, and surrounding yourself with supportive people as key factors in maintaining a healthy weight long-term.